Criteria for Selecting the Leading Health Indicators for *Healthy People 2030*

Committee on Informing the Selection of
Leading Health Indicators for *Healthy People 2030*

Board on Population Health and Public Health Practice

Health and Medicine Division

A Consensus Study Report of

The National Academies of
SCIENCES · ENGINEERING · MEDICINE

THE NATIONAL ACADEMIES PRESS
Washington, DC
www.nap.edu

THE NATIONAL ACADEMIES PRESS 500 Fifth Street, NW Washington, DC 20001

This activity was supported by a contract between the National Academy of Sciences and the Department of Health and Human Services (HHSP233201400020B). Any opinions, findings, conclusions, or recommendations expressed in this publication do not necessarily reflect the views of any organization or agency that provided support for the project.

International Standard Book Number-13: 978-0-309-49594-3
International Standard Book Number-10: 0-309-49594-6
Digital Object Identifier: https://doi.org/10.17226/25531

Additional copies of this publication are available from the National Academies Press, 500 Fifth Street, NW, Keck 360, Washington, DC 20001; (800) 624-6242 or (202) 334-3313; http://www.nap.edu.

Printed in the United States of America

Suggested citation: National Academies of Sciences, Engineering, and Medicine. 2019. *Criteria for selecting the Leading Health Indicators for* Healthy People 2030. Washington, DC: The National Academies Press. https://doi.org/10.17226/25531.

The National Academies of

SCIENCES · ENGINEERING · MEDICINE

The **National Academy of Sciences** was established in 1863 by an Act of Congress, signed by President Lincoln, as a private, nongovernmental institution to advise the nation on issues related to science and technology. Members are elected by their peers for outstanding contributions to research. Dr. Marcia McNutt is president.

The **National Academy of Engineering** was established in 1964 under the charter of the National Academy of Sciences to bring the practices of engineering to advising the nation. Members are elected by their peers for extraordinary contributions to engineering. Dr. John L. Anderson is president.

The **National Academy of Medicine** (formerly the Institute of Medicine) was established in 1970 under the charter of the National Academy of Sciences to advise the nation on medical and health issues. Members are elected by their peers for distinguished contributions to medicine and health. Dr. Victor J. Dzau is president.

The three Academies work together as the **National Academies of Sciences, Engineering, and Medicine** to provide independent, objective analysis and advice to the nation and conduct other activities to solve complex problems and inform public policy decisions. The National Academies also encourage education and research, recognize outstanding contributions to knowledge, and increase public understanding in matters of science, engineering, and medicine.

Learn more about the National Academies of Sciences, Engineering, and Medicine at **www.nationalacademies.org**.

The National Academies of
SCIENCES • ENGINEERING • MEDICINE

COMMITTEE ON INFORMING THE SELECTION OF LEADING HEALTH INDICATORS FOR *HEALTHY PEOPLE 2030*

GEORGE J. ISHAM (*Chair*), Senior Fellow, HealthPartners Institute
EBONY BOULWARE, Professor of Medicine; Chief, Division of General Internal Medicine; Vice Dean, Translational Science; Associate Vice Chancellor, Translational Research, Duke University School of Medicine
GILBERT GEE, Professor, Department of Community Health Sciences, UCLA Fielding School of Public Health, University of California, Los Angeles
MARTHE R. GOLD, Senior Scholar, The New York Academy of Medicine
SHERI JOHNSON, Director, Population Health Institute, Associate Professor, Department of Population Health Sciences, University of Wisconsin–Madison, School of Medicine and Public Health
PAULA LANTZ, Associate Dean for Academic Affairs, Professor of Public Policy, Gerald R. Ford School of Public Policy, University of Michigan
DARCY PHELAN-EMRICK, Chief Epidemiologist, Baltimore City Health Department; Assistant Scientist, Johns Hopkins Bloomberg School of Public Health
JONATHAN S. SKINNER, James O. Freedman Presidential Professor in Economics, Department of Economics, Dartmouth Institute for Health Policy and Clinical Practice, Geisel School of Medicine, Dartmouth College

Study Staff

ALINA B. BACIU, Study Director
CARLA S. ALVARADO, Program Officer
ANNA W. MARTIN, Administrative Assistant
ROSE MARIE MARTINEZ, Senior Director, Board on Population Health and Public Health Practice

Reviewers

This Consensus Study Report was reviewed in draft form by individuals chosen for their diverse perspectives and technical expertise. The purpose of this independent review is to provide candid and critical comments that will assist the National Academies of Sciences, Engineering, and Medicine in making each published report as sound as possible and to ensure that it meets the institutional standards for quality, objectivity, evidence, and responsiveness to the study charge. The review comments and draft manuscript remain confidential to protect the integrity of the deliberative process.

We thank the following individuals for their review of this report:

JOHN AUERBACH, Trust for America's Health
ANA DIEZ ROUX, Drexel University
CYNTHIA HAQ, University of California, Irvine
JOSÉ A. PAGAN, New York University
STEVEN M. TEUTSCH, Public Health Institute and University of California, Los Angeles

Although the reviewers listed above provided many constructive comments and suggestions, they were not asked to endorse the conclusions or recommendations of this report nor did they see the final draft before its release. The review of this report was overseen by **ERIC B. LARSON,** Kaiser Permanente Washington, and **JAMES S. HOUSE,** University of Michigan. They were responsible for making certain that an independent examination of this report was carried out in accordance with the standards of the National Academies and that all review comments were carefully considered. Responsibility for the final content rests entirely with the authoring committee and the National Academies.

Acknowledgments

The committee wishes to thank and acknowledge the many individuals and organizations that contributed to the study process and development of this report.

The committee appreciates the opportunity to assist the Department of Health and Human Services by providing advice on a key aspect of its *Healthy People 2030* effort.

The committee is grateful to experts who informed its deliberations through presentations and discussions that took place at the committee's public meetings. Several individuals provided background and insights about the Secretary's Advisory Committee on National Health Promotion and Disease Prevention Objectives for 2030 (SAC)—they included Deputy Assistant Secretary for Health Donald Wright, director of the Office of Disease Prevention and Health Promotion (ODPHP) Carter Blakey, ODPHP staff member Tiffani Kigenyi, SAC co-chairs Dushanka Kleinman and Nico Pronk, and subcommittee chairs Therese Richmond and Edward Sondik. Other speakers included Anita Chandra, Tom Eckstein, Marjory Givens, Kristen Lewis, Bobby Milstein, Ali Mokdad, Amy O'Hara, Carley Riley, Brian Smedley, Soma Stout, Sarah Treuhaft, and Steven Woolf.[1]

The committee thanks the National Academies of Sciences, Engineering, and Medicine staff who contributed to the production of this report, including study staff Alina Baciu, Carla Alvarado, Anna Martin, and Rose Marie Martinez. The committee's work received additional research support from Andrew Koltun, Georgetown University medical student and

[1] Steven Woolf's slides were presented by Brian Smedley at the May 28, 2019, meeting.

population health scholar, who completed his summer practicum in the Health and Medicine Division (HMD). This project received assistance from Misrak Dabi (Office of Financial Administration); Clyde Behney, Lauren Shern, and Taryn Young (HMD Executive Office); and HMD communications staff, including Jeanay Butler, Sadaf Faraz, and Tina Seliber.

Finally, the National Academies staff offers thanks to the executive assistants of committee members who provided scheduling support: Nancy Langer and Harriet Ware.

Contents

Acronyms and Abbreviations

FIW	Federal Interagency Workgroup
HHS	Department of Health and Human Services
HP2030/2020/2010	*Healthy People 2030/2020/2010*
IOM	Institute of Medicine
LHI	Leading Health Indicator
OMH	HHS Office of Minority Health
SAC	Secretary's Advisory Committee on National Health Promotion and Disease Prevention Objectives for 2030

Summary

The Assistant Secretary for Health has charged this National Academies of Sciences, Engineering, and Medicine committee with assisting

> in the development of Leading Health Indicators (LHIs) for *Healthy People 2030*. The committee will develop (1) recommendations regarding the criteria for selecting LHIs and (2) a slate of LHIs that will serve as options for the Healthy People Federal Interagency Workgroup to consider as they develop the final criteria and set of LHIs for *Healthy People 2030*. The committee may identify gaps and may recommend new objectives for LHI consideration that meet the core objective criteria.

This brief report responds to the first part of the task. The committee reviewed past and current Healthy People materials, both those developed by the Department of Health and Human Services (HHS) and the current Secretary's Advisory Committee on National Health Promotion and Disease Prevention Objectives for 2030 (SAC), and prior National Academies reports. The committee's information-gathering activities included three open meetings: two were online and consisted of presentations from HHS and the leadership of the SAC and its relevant subcommittees, and one meeting took place at the Keck Center of the National Academies in Washington, DC.

In this report, the committee makes four findings and two recommendations based on its review of relevant materials and information.

Finding 1: The committee finds that the *Healthy People 2030* draft objectives document is missing some key topics necessary to fully reflect the intent of the *Healthy People 2030* Framework's vision, mission, foundational principles, and overarching goals.[1]

Finding 2: The committee finds that the draft objectives do not offer an appropriately balanced and comprehensive range from which to derive Leading Health Indicators that also reflect the intent of the *Healthy People 2030* Framework's vision, mission, foundational principles, and overarching goals.

Finding 3: The committee finds that the *Healthy People 2030* draft objectives document includes too few objectives that allow for making important comparisons to other countries, including to peer nations in the Organisation for Economic Co-operation and Development.

Finding 4: The committee finds that if the existing criteria for Leading Health Indicator (LHI) selection were applied to the existing *Healthy People 2030* draft objectives, the resulting LHI set would not be aligned with the *Healthy People 2030* Framework—it would not tell a coherent story about the nation's (or communities') health, well-being, and the state of health equity.

Recommendation 1: The committee recommends that the Department of Health and Human Services and the Federal Interagency Workgroup add to the *Healthy People 2030* objectives topics or implement a structural reorganization (with additional topics) that will yield more core objectives that reflect the *Healthy People 2030* Framework and could lead to better Leading Health Indicators. Cross-cutting topics (i.e., topics that refer to or link with multiple health states, life stages, systems, and all dimensions of health) should include health equity; the social, physical, and economic determinants of health; shared responsibility and multiple sectors; and all levels of government.

Recommendation 2: The committee recommends a three-phase process should be used for Leading Health Indicator (LHI) selection from the *Healthy People 2030* objectives. A new phase would precede the existing two, and it would apply the *Healthy People 2030*

[1] Refers to the topic categories under which lists of objectives are nested beginning with Adolescent Health and concluding with Vision.

Framework (especially the vision, mission, foundational principles, and overarching goals) in consideration of additional objectives and in selecting LHIs.

1

Introduction

At the request of the Department of Health and Human Services' (HHS's) Office of the Assistant Secretary for Health, the National Academies of Sciences, Engineering, and Medicine appointed a committee of experts to assist HHS with one component of the Healthy People initiative. Healthy People is a decadal HHS effort launched in 1979 to "develop a framework for improving the health of all people in the United States" and offer "a strategic agenda to align health promotion and disease prevention activities in communities around the country" (Azar, 2018). The National Academies committee was given the following Statement of Task:

> The Department of Health and Human Services, Office of the Assistant Secretary for Health, requests that the National Academies of Sciences, Engineering, and Medicine convene an ad hoc committee to assist in the development of Leading Health Indicators (LHIs) for *Healthy People 2030*. The committee will develop (1) recommendations regarding the criteria for selecting LHIs and (2) a slate of LHIs that will serve as options for the Healthy People Federal Interagency Workgroup to consider as they develop the final criteria and set of LHIs for *Healthy People 2030*. The committee may identify gaps and may recommend new objectives for LHI consideration that meet the core objective criteria.

This brief report represents the National Academies committee (or "the committee") response to the first portion of the charge, providing a review of the criteria for selecting LHIs along with—in response to the last sentence of the charge—comments about the *Healthy People 2030* objectives (HP2030 objectives), currently in draft form. This report lays the groundwork for the second report, which will provide additional comments about the HP2030 objectives from which LHIs are to be selected, and will recommend a slate of LHIs.

At the time the National Academies committee began its work in late 2018, the Secretary's Advisory Committee on National Health Promotion and Disease Prevention Objectives for 2030 (SAC) had met 12 times and had developed the framework for *Healthy People 2030* (HP2030 Framework) incorporating a round of public comments. The SAC has prepared seven reports, on topics including the criteria for selecting the HP2030 objectives and the criteria for selecting the LHIs, and the SAC also worked with outside experts to prepare a series of briefs intended to "clarify, discuss, and offer insights" about the HP2030 Framework (see Box 1-1 for the Framework) (SAC, 2019a). By late 2018, the Federal Interagency Workgroup (FIW), which includes HHS agencies and representatives of other federal departments, had also met to generate the HP2030 objectives, which were expected to be aligned with the HP2030 Framework. The draft objectives were released for public comment between December 2018 and January 2019.

Because the HP2030 objectives will not be finalized and released until 2020, the National Academies committee was asked to first comment on the draft LHI criteria and then, in preparation for its second report proposing a set of LHIs to inform the work of the FIW, review the objectives and identify relevant gaps in the core objectives in accordance with the core objective criteria. Figure 1-1 describes the main inputs and timeline for the LHIs for *Healthy People 2030*.

BOX 1-1
***Healthy People 2030* Framework:**
Vision, Mission, Principles, Goals[a]
(developed by the Secretary's Advisory Committee)

Vision: A society in which all people can achieve their full potential for health and well-being across the life span.

Mission: To promote, strengthen, and evaluate the nation's efforts to improve the health and well-being of all people.

BOX 1-1 Continued

Foundational principles: Foundational principles explain the thinking that guides decisions about *Healthy People 2030.* The health and well-being of all people and communities are essential to a thriving, equitable society. Promoting health and well-being and preventing disease are linked efforts that encompass physical, mental, and social health dimensions. Investing to achieve the full potential for health and well-being for all provides valuable benefits to society. Achieving health and well-being requires eliminating health disparities, achieving health equity, and attaining health literacy. Healthy physical, social, and economic environments strengthen the potential to achieve health and well-being. Promoting and achieving the nation's health and well-being is a shared responsibility that is distributed across the national, state, tribal, and community levels, including the public, private, and not-for-profit sectors. Working to attain the full potential for health and well-being of the population is a component of decision making and policy formulation across all sectors.

Overarching goals: Attain healthy, thriving lives and well-being, free of preventable disease, disability, injury, and premature death. Eliminate health disparities, achieve health equity, and attain health literacy to improve the health and well-being of all. Create social, physical, and economic environments that promote attaining full potential for health and well-being for all. Promote healthy development, healthy behaviors, and well-being across all life stages. Engage leadership, key constituents, and the public across multiple sectors to take action and design policies that improve the health and well-being of all.

Plan of action: Set national goals and measurable objectives to guide evidence-based policies, programs, and other actions to improve health and well-being. Provide data that are accurate, timely, accessible, and can drive targeted actions to address regions and populations with poor health or at high risk for poor health in the future. Foster improvement through public and private efforts to improve health and well-being for people of all ages and the communities in which they live. Provide tools for the public, programs, policy makers, and others to evaluate progress toward improving health and well-being. Share and support the implementation of evidence-based programs and policies that are replicable, scalable, and sustainable. Report biennially on progress throughout the decade from 2020 to 2030. Stimulate research and innovation toward meeting *Healthy People 2030* goals and highlight critical research, data, and evaluation needs. Facilitate development and availability of affordable means of health promotion, disease prevention, and treatment.

NOTE: The Healthy People Framework includes a preamble that summarizes the background, history, and contributions of the Healthy People initiative.

[a] See https://www.healthypeople.gov/2020/About-Healthy-People/Development-Healthy-People-2030/Framework (accessed July 9, 2019).

SOURCE: HHS, 2019a.

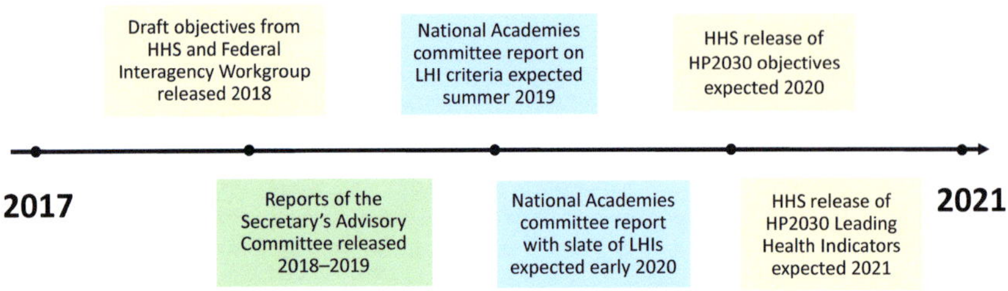

FIGURE 1-1 Main inputs into and timeline for the selection of Leading Health Indicators by the Department of Health and Human Services and the Federal Interagency Workgroup.
NOTE: HHS = Department of Health and Human Services; HP2030 = *Healthy People 2030*; LHI = Leading Health Indicator.

REFLECTIONS ON THE HP2030 FRAMEWORK

The SAC's *Recommendations for the* Healthy People 2030 *Leading Health Indicators* (2018a) described the HP2030 Framework as "a foundation for the criteria for selecting LHIs for the *Healthy People 2030* initiative." In the same report, the SAC stated that it was proposing "criteria for selecting *Healthy People* 2030 LHIs that are informed by the *Healthy People* 2030 Framework,[1] including the vision, mission, foundational principles, overarching goals, and plan of action."

The National Academies committee recognizes that the HP2030 Framework has built considerably on the foundation of previous Healthy People efforts by broadening the conceptual framing of the initiative to strengthen the emphasis on health equity; expand the consideration of the social, environmental, and economic determinants of health; and add the useful and multidimensional notion of well-being. This evolution of the HP2030 Framework is consistent with recent advances in the understanding of those factors that lead to better health and well-being, and the set of issue briefs released by the SAC provides context and the evidence base for the main elements of the Framework (SAC, 2019a). Below, the National Academies committee further discusses the relevance of the major elements of the HP2030 Framework to the HP2030 objectives and LHIs:

- The health equity focus of the Framework underscores the importance of disaggregating information, when feasible, about the LHIs by race, ethnicity, rurality, and other characteristics.

[1] Underline added for emphasis.

However, this is not enough. Measures of health equity are also needed. In defining health equity as "the principle underlying a commitment to reduce—and, ultimately, eliminate—disparities in health and in its determinants, including social determinants," Braveman (2014) referred to *Healthy People 2020* as the first time that a federal government entity defined health disparity with specificity. *Healthy People 2020* described disparities as "linked with economic, social, or environmental disadvantage" or with other "characteristics historically linked to discrimination or exclusion" (SAC, 2010). Braveman added to the definition that "pursuing health equity means striving for the highest possible standard of health for all people and giving special attention to the needs of those at greatest risk of poor health, based on social conditions" (Braveman, 2014).

- The determinants of health focus calls for both acknowledging the evidence showing those factors account for the largest effect on health outcomes, and highlighting the value of a cross-sector and all-levels-of-government approach to health promotion.
- The well-being focus is consonant with the longstanding World Health Organization definition of health and its physical, mental, and social dimensions (WHO, 2014), and it offers a further link for engaging the attention of sectors that make important contributions to population well-being, for exploring the metrics available from those other sectors, and for comparing against what other countries measure. A key aspect of this focus is that health is not simply the absence of disease or injury; it is also related to being well in social and emotional terms.

2

Past Selection Criteria Described for the Leading Health Indicators and Other High-Level Indicator Sets

The National Academies of Sciences, Engineering, and Medicine committee reviewed several relevant sets of criteria developed by the Department of Health and Human Services and in previous National Academies reports that were intended to guide the selection of past Leading Health Indicators (LHIs) or other concise and high-level sets of national indicators. The following sections describe the committee's thinking regarding these sets of criteria.

In the *Healthy People 2010* initiative, the LHIs were defined as

> a subset of the *Healthy People 2010* objectives that reflect the major public health concerns in the United States ... chosen on the basis of their ability to motivate action, the availability of data to measure their progress, and their relevance as broad public health issues. These indicators reflect individual behaviors, physical and social environmental factors, and important health system issues that greatly affect the health of individuals and communities. (NCHS, 2010, LHI-3)

Although the National Academies committee could not locate a list of criteria for *Healthy People 2020* LHI selection, it noted the following about LHIs for *Healthy People 2020*:

> [The LHIs were] selected and organized using a Health Determinants and Health Outcomes by Life Stages conceptual framework. This approach is intended to draw attention to both individual and societal determinants that affect the public's health and contribute to health disparities from

infancy through old age, thereby highlighting strategic opportunities to promote health and improve quality of life for all Americans.

Determinants of Health and Health Disparities. Biological, social, economic, and environmental factors—and their interrelationships—influence the ability of individuals and communities to make progress on these indicators. Addressing these determinants is key to improving population health, eliminating health disparities, and meeting the overarching goals of *Healthy People 2020*.

Health Across Life Stages. LHIs are being examined using a life stages perspective. This approach recognizes that specific risk factors and determinants of health vary across the life span. Health and disease result from the accumulation (over time) of the effects of risk factors and determinants. Intervening at specific points in the life course can help reduce risk factors and promote health. The life-stages perspective addresses one of the four overarching goals of *Healthy People 2020*: "Promote quality life, healthy development, and health behaviors across all life stages" (HHS, 2019b).

The Institute of Medicine (IOM) 1999 report *Leading Health Indicators for* Healthy People 2010 recommended six criteria for LHIs:

1. worth measuring;
2. can be measured for diverse populations;
3. understood by people who need to act;
4. information will galvanize action;
5. actions that can lead to improvement are known and feasible; and
6. measurement over time will reflect results of action (IOM, 1999).

The 2011 IOM report *Leading Health Indicators for* Healthy People 2020 added three criteria to the 1999 list: (1) the objective is well defined; (2) data for the objective are available for various geographic levels (local, national) and population subgroups (e.g., race/ethnic, socioeconomic status, rural/urban); and (3) changes in societal domains other than health (e.g., socioeconomic or environmental conditions or public policies) can have a detectable effect on the objective (IOM, 2011).

The 2015 IOM report *Vital Signs: Core Metrics for Health and Health Care Progress* outlined criteria for a small set of national measures. The criteria for selecting individual core measures were "importance for health, strength of linkage to progress, understandability of the measure, technical integrity, potential for broader system impact, and utility at multiple levels." Criteria for the set were "systemic reach, outcomes-oriented, person meaningful, parsimonious, representative, [and] utility at multiple levels" (IOM, 2015, p. 14).

The 2013 IOM report *Toward Quality Measures for Population Health and the Leading Health Indicators* stated that criteria for conditions or outcomes to be measured should be "reflective of a high preventable burden and actionable at the appropriate level for intervention." The report gave the following criteria for measures under consideration:

- Timely—data collection frequency and timeliness of availability;
- Usable for assessing various populations (zip code, different levels of government, etc.);
- Understandable (includes face validity, transparency);
- Methodologically rigorous (having suitable methodological and quantitative characteristics, such as sensitivity, specificity, reliability, validity, and consistency over time, and being managed by an established, regularly updated process); and
- Accepted and harmonized (e.g., endorsed by the National Quality Forum or used by America's Health Rankings or County Health Rankings) (IOM, 2013).

The 2010 IOM report *For the Public's Health: The Role of Measurement in Action and Accountability* put forward the following criteria:

- Face validity (meaningfulness, relevance, and understandability),
- Feasibility (availability or collectability of data),
- Methodologic soundness (validity and reliability), and
- Fairness (to the stakeholders whose performance they will evaluate).

3

The *Healthy People 2030* Draft Objectives

ABOUT THE *HEALTHY PEOPLE 2030* DRAFT OBJECTIVES AND RELEVANCE FOR LEADING HEALTH INDICATORS (LHIs)

The Secretary's Advisory Committee on National Health Promotion and Disease Prevention Objectives for 2030 (SAC) has defined the LHIs as "a selected set of measures of determinants and sentinel indicators of current and potential changes in population health and well-being" that "*will be drawn from Healthy People objectives* to communicate the highest-priority health issues."[1] Moreover, "The set of LHIs should contain a small number of objectives" and "enough LHIs should be included in that set to focus attention and drive action on top health priorities" (SAC, 2018a).

The *Healthy People 2030* (HP2030) draft objectives prepared by the Department of Health and Human Services (HHS) and the Federal Interagency Workgroup (FIW) are divided into three categories: core, research, and developmental. These are defined in Box 3-1. The core objectives will provide the basis for selecting the LHIs, as described in the SAC's *Recommendations for the Healthy People 2030 Leading Health Indicators* (2018a).

To inform its work, the National Academies of Sciences, Engineering, and Medicine committee reviewed all seven extant SAC reports,[2] including *Report on* Healthy People 2030 *Leading Health Indicators* and Report 7, *Assessment and Recommendations for Proposed Objectives for* Healthy People 2030. Because the LHI selection criteria begin with "[a]ll core objectives,"

---

[1] Italics added for emphasis.

[2] All reports are available at https://www.healthypeople.gov/2020/About-Healthy-People/Development-Healthy-People-2030/Committee-Meetings (accessed June 21, 2019).

BOX 3-1
Types of Objectives for *Healthy People 2030* (developed by the Secretary's Advisory Committee on National Health Promotion and Disease Prevention Objectives for 2030)

Healthy People 2030 will include three distinct types of objectives:

1. *Core objectives:* Core objectives are the central component of *Healthy People 2030*. These are measurable objectives for which a 2030 target will be set. Core objectives are the high-priority public health issues that when addressed, will improve our nation's health. Core objectives must have (1) an identified and approved data source, (2) baseline data using data no older than 2015 and a measure of variability if applicable (for example, if the data source is a sample survey), and (3) assurance of at least two additional data points throughout the decade. Additionally, (4) evidence-based interventions should be identified for core objectives.
2. *Developmental objectives:* Developmental objectives represent high priority issues that do not yet have the reliable baseline data needed to make them core objectives. Evidence-based interventions have been identified for developmental objectives.
3. *Research objectives:* Research objectives represent key opportunities to make progress in areas where there has been limited research to date, but where the health or economic burden is high or evidence shows significant disparities between population groups. Research objectives may or may not meet core objective data requirements, and do not yet have evidence-based interventions developed. Research objectives will vary in scope and specificity, and might also be considered priority areas for future research or emerging issues.

NOTES: Developmental and research objectives that meet the core objective selection criteria before 2030 may be considered for inclusion in the *Healthy People 2030* core during the decade. However, there is no guarantee that developmental and research objectives will become core objectives even once they meet the criteria.
SOURCE: SAC, 2018.

the National Academies committee also reviewed the HP2030 draft objectives available on the HHS Healthy People website and the objective selection criteria (see Box 3-1) to understand the material from which the LHIs are intended to be drawn (HHS, 2019b).[3]

[3] The HP2030 draft objectives posted for public comment between December 2018 and January 2019 are available at https://www.healthypeople.gov/sites/default/files/ObjectivesPublicComment508_1.17.19.pdf (accessed June 20, 2019).

COMMENTS ON THE CRITERIA FOR SELECTING *HEALTHY PEOPLE 2030* OBJECTIVES

The National Academies committee agrees with the five criteria described by the SAC for selecting the HP2030 objectives, two of which are specific to core objectives (see Box 3-2). Below, the committee clarifies its interpretation of criteria 2, 4, and 5 in anticipation of proposing in its second report new core objectives that may be necessary for some of the LHIs.

With respect to the need for criterion 2, current baseline data, the National Academies committee suggests that the FIW and the Secretary of HHS consider the use of new data sources when indicators that track needs related to critical health and well-being are unavailable. These may include other sources of federal data-gathering efforts (e.g., in the Department of Housing and Urban Development and the Department of Transportation), as well as comparably rigorous data from private entities (e.g., Gallup Well-Being Index) and from large external data sets such as those made possible by "big data." Although reliance on many types of data sources, whether public or private, may be affected by a level of uncertainty about a source's quality and sustainability over time, it is likely a federal agency could support continuing an especially valuable data source. (The HP2030 draft objectives include a narrow subset of data sources from other federal agencies, such as the Department of Agriculture data pertaining to food security and the Department of Education data pertaining to educational milestones and to disability.) In all cases where new objectives are identified, the data sources from which they are gathered would need to conform to the same stringent quality review as do those currently in use.

With respect to criterion 4, evidence, the committee notes that the LHIs are to be drawn from core objectives (those in the current draft that will remain in the final HP2030 objectives as well as newly added items). The committee underscores the need to accommodate levels of evidence appropriate to the domain, time frame, and type of intervention in assessing the adequacy of evidence emerging from interventions conducted by other sectors that address upstream drivers of health and well-being. This approach would allow for the inclusion of a broad range of interventions that address food, shelter, climate change threats and resiliency, education, transportation, built environment, and economic security, recognizing that these are prerequisites for health and well-being. Although in principle, all population health interventions will be based on the highest level of evidence, studying the effects of policy and regulatory interventions outside of health and medical care can be extraordinarily challenging. Evaluation of the effect of these interventions is complicated

BOX 3-2
Criteria for the *Healthy People 2030* (HP2030) Objectives (developed by the Secretary's Advisory Committee on National Health Promotion and Disease Prevention Objectives for 2030)

1. **Measurable.** The core objective must be measurable by the data cutoff for inclusion in HP2030, which is mid-2019.
2. **Current Baseline Data.** The core objective must reasonably be expected to have a baseline using data no older than 2015, and at least 2 additional data points during the HP2030 decade.
3. **National Importance.** The objective must be of national importance. To meet the "national importance" criterion, objectives should have a direct impact or influence on health, broad and comprehensive applicability, a substantial burden, and they should address a national health priority.

   a. Direct impact or influence on health: Does this objective address an outcome or preventive/risk factor that has a direct impact on population health?
   b. Broad and comprehensive applicability: Does this objective address a broad health concern or topic that is applicable to a large part of the population, as opposed to being limited to more narrowly defined groups?
   c. Substantial burden: Does this objective address a health concern that represents a substantial impact or potential impact on the health or well-being of an individual or on a population?
   d. National (not just federal) public health priority: Does this objective address a public health priority of the Department of Health and Human Services, national prevention initiatives, other national indicator projects, and efforts at the state, local, and tribal level across the country?

by (1) the fact that all populations in a region would be exposed (and may benefit to lesser and greater extents), (2) the myriad outcomes they are intended to address (not all directly health related), (3) the typically long time frame required to analyze policy effectiveness, and (4) the paucity of resources that are available to evaluate outcomes. The effect of interventions at the policy level may often be first, and perhaps only, understood through observational studies and natural experiments. The committee believes that this type of evidence is valid and useful in the policy context, and it may work to ensure that more upstream objectives—that reflect the HP2030 Framework—are identified.

The committee reviewed a number of documents and presentations that the FIW references in its definition of effectiveness as it pertains to

4. **Evidence-Base.** The objective should have a known evidence-base, and identified evidence-based interventions to improve outcomes. The effectiveness of the objectives was rated based on the scale used in *Healthy People 2020* to rate evidence-based resources on the website.
5. **Health Equity and Disparities.** The objectives should address health disparities and/or support achieving health equity. Health equity and disparities have been an important part of the Healthy People initiative since *Healthy People 2000*. Health equity is defined by the Department of Health and Human Services' Office of Minority Health (OMH) as, "Attainment of the highest level of health for all people. Achieving health equity requires valuing everyone equally with focused and ongoing societal efforts to address avoidable inequalities, historical and contemporary injustices, and the elimination of health and healthcare disparities." OMH defines health disparities as, "A particular type of health difference that is closely linked with social or economic disadvantage. Health disparities adversely affect groups of people who have systematically experienced greater social and/or economic obstacles to health and/or a clean environment based on their racial or ethnic group; religion; socioeconomic status; gender; age; mental health; cognitive, sensory, or physical disability; sexual orientation; geographic location; or other characteristics historically linked to discrimination or exclusion." Objectives are also considered for inclusion, based on the expectation that the data source is able to track the following population level data.

   - Sex
   - Race/Ethnicity
   - Age
   - Educational Attainment
   - Family Income
   - Health Insurance Status
   - Geographic Location or Region
   - Marital Status
   - Sexual Orientation
   - Gender Identity
   - Disability Status

SOURCE: SAC, 2018b.

core objectives. The *Healthy People 2020* process rated evidence on a scale of 1–4, with the highest level (4, rigorous) described as that emerging from recommendations of the U.S. Preventive Services Task Force, the Community Preventive Services Task Force, or systematic reviews published in peer-reviewed journals. Level 3, or "strong" evidence, rests on nonsystematic reviews published by the federal government and nonsystematic reviews published in peer-reviewed journals. Level 2, seen as "moderate" evidence, emerges from journal articles of individual studies, published intervention research, and published pilot studies. Level 1, regarded as "weak," lists intervention evaluations or "studies without peer review that have evidence of effectiveness, feasibility, reach, sustainability, and transferability" (HHS, n.d.). The committee recognizes the tension inherent in broadening the framework of considerations of health and well-being at the same time that *Healthy People 2030* seeks to promote and adhere to high standards of evidence for intervention effectiveness. It is the committee's view that in seeking LHIs that best represent high-level priorities for the nation, it will be important to maintain accommodation of levels of evidence appropriate to the domain, time frame, and type of intervention with respect to what constitutes evidence adequacy when drawing from work conducted in other sectors. This view resonates with the *Healthy People 2020* publication *Evidence-Based Clinical and Public Health: Generating and Applying the Evidence*, which discusses the "limitations of the traditional hierarchy of evidence" and "the need for contextual information" (SAC, 2010, p. 11). That report acknowledges that "many public health interventions are not amenable to randomized trials" because of their "complexity and interdisciplinary nature," but the report notes that many other types of analyses "can provide a rigorous assessment that can justify a broad recommendation." As one example, the report describes health impact assessment as a tool for evaluating the effects on health of policies in other sectors (SAC, 2010).

With regard to contributions from other sectors, the National Academies committee notes with appreciation that the SAC meetings included discussion about the role of other sectors on several occasions. For example, the ninth meeting of the SAC in May 2018 included an update about the FIW efforts to generate HP2030 draft objectives. A member of the SAC asked how the FIW plans to engage nontraditional health sectors (e.g., agriculture, education, transportation) in the selection of objectives and the development of *Healthy People 2030*. The FIW representative responded that the group includes representatives from every federal department (HHS, 2018). The cross-sectoral connections implicit in creating well-being also were acknowledged at the eighth meeting of the SAC in February 2018, where one member noted that the FIW "has worked diligently to build bridges between different sectors and agencies, particularly among those with data who might not consider themselves as typically included in the health sector." A co-chair of the SAC added, "Other sectors and partners may be more receptive to language about improving well-being rather than health, and that their data sources could be viewed through this lens." For example, decision makers in transportation might not think of their work as directed toward improving health, but the notion of enhancing the well-being of people and communities may resonate with concepts familiar to them, such as livability and quality of life.[4]

[4] Summary of the February 28, 2019, Meeting of the Secretary's Advisory Committee can be found at https://www.healthypeople.gov/sites/default/files/Feb_28_2018_Meeting%20 Summary_Secretary-s_Advisory_Committee_for_2030_1.pdf (accessed June 25, 2019).

Criterion 5, health equity and disparities, outlines the many social and economic factors that have created or contributed to current inequities in health and well-being. The committee notes the listing of the many subpopulations that continue to experience unjustly disparate levels of health (Braveman, 2014). In the selection of candidate LHIs, the committee recognizes that not all LHIs will demonstrate inequities for all listed subpopulations, the detraction from health and well-being may be systematically greater for certain subpopulations, and limitations on data availability may make disaggregation difficult to achieve for all indicators. The committee believes that at minimum, all LHIs need to track progress on the basis of educational attainment, race, ethnicity, income or wealth (or equivalent), and geographic location, primarily urban versus rural.

COMMENTS ON THE HP2030 DRAFT OBJECTIVES

Clearly, the HP2030 draft objectives[5] represent a broad range of topics (from "Adolescent Health" to "Vision") and reflect issues of importance to a wide community of stakeholders in the public and private sectors. However, on its review of the more than 350 draft core objectives for their suitability as potential LHIs, the committee made four findings.

> **Finding 1:** The committee finds that the *Healthy People 2030* draft objectives document is missing some key topics necessary to fully reflect the intent of the *Healthy People 2030* Framework's vision, mission, foundational principles, and overarching goals.[6]

The draft topics and the objectives nested in each topic demonstrate a disconnection from the aspirations of the HP2030 process reflected in the Framework and the explanatory issue briefs. The key words of the HP2030 Framework include *health equity; well-being; social, physical, and economic determinants of health; shared responsibility and [the roles for] multiple sectors, all levels of government; all life stages;* and *all dimensions of health* (i.e., physical, mental, and social). The 41 HP2030 topics under which the 355 draft core objectives (and additional research and developmental objectives) are organized could be classified as follows, in order of prevalence: health states (approximately 14 that primarily pertain to health states),

[5] The HP2030 draft objectives released by HHS for public comment in December 3, 2018, to January 17, 2019, are available at https://www.healthypeople.gov/sites/default/files/ObjectivesPublicComment508_1.17.19.pdf (accessed June 19, 2019).

[6] See Box 1-1 for the vision, mission, foundational principles, and goals of the HP2030 Framework (or Appendix E for the complete Framework).

systems (approximately 10 that primarily pertain to systems), life stages, and the social, physical, and economic determinants of health. The social determinants of health are primarily organized in one eponymous topic area, with a small number in two to three additional topic areas, but they are not shown and do not operate as a cross-cutting topic, such as social determinants of health that apply to different life stages, or with systematic attention to upstream factors that are linked with several different health states or outcomes. Having topics and objectives that are explicitly aligned with the concept of well-being is not only consistent with the ecological model of health, but it may also help explain the importance of cross-sector coordination and collaboration, and "shared responsibility." This is articulated in the foundational principles of the HP2030 Framework, which state "[h]ealthy physical, social, and economic environments strengthen the potential to achieve health and well-being" and "[p]romoting and achieving the nation's health and well-being is a shared responsibility that is distributed across the national, state, tribal, and community levels, including the public, private, and not-for-profit sectors."

The misalignment of draft objectives with the HP2030 Framework may be a result of the two different processes involved in (1) developing the HP2030 Framework and (2) generating the HP2030 draft objectives. The process of developing the HP2030 Framework was a top-down or big-picture process that sought to provide the high-level parameters for the nation's path toward equitable health and well-being. In contrast, the objective development process was a bottom-up nominal process that gathered draft objectives from three work streams of the Federal Interagency Workgroup and 42 HP2020 topic-specific workgroups (HHS, 2018). Workgroups were instructed to reduce the number of objectives compared to *Healthy People 2020* (from more than 1,200 to approximately 375). This process appeared to emphasize a continuity of topics and objectives from the past decade's Healthy People effort, which might be a primary reason the objectives do not fully represent the ideas of the HP2030 Framework. It also is unclear whether the FIW workgroups generating and vetting objectives were explicitly asked to consider what would make good LHIs and include such objectives in their contributions.

Finding 2: The committee finds that the draft objectives do not offer an appropriately balanced and comprehensive range from which to derive Leading Health Indicators that also reflect the intent of the *Healthy People 2030* Framework's vision, mission, foundational principles, and overarching goals.

As noted above, a major change to *Healthy People 2030* is the emphasis on well-being and the determinants of health and well-being. There are important objectives that lack a focus "across all life stages" (one of the overarching goals in the HP2030 Framework); for example, child poverty has been discarded, and only an overall measure of poverty remains. Health measures specific to children are leading indicators of future national health in 2030 and for decades to come, yet few objectives address, for example, the proportion of children with access to effective early intervention programs.[7] One possible way to disaggregate a larger objective or to consolidate many fragmented objectives would be to develop some objectives that have sub-objectives (see, for example, the proposal in IOM, 2011, starting on p. 77). Examples could include an objective on poverty with sub-objectives for child poverty, poverty among older adults, and poverty in specific categories of race/ethnicity, or an objective on foodborne illness with sub-objectives for specific foodborne illnesses, such as those currently listed under the food safety topic of the current HP2030 draft objectives.

The six core objectives under the social determinants of health topic of the HP2030 draft objectives represent a disparate assortment that includes two objectives related to employment, two on education, one on housing, and one on incarceration and criminal justice. A more systematic approach to each of the social, physical, and economic determinants of health—as described in the HP2030 Framework and in the issue briefs—would consider all areas where the evidence is robust or strong, as well as linkages with life stages, among other cross-cutting considerations. For example, the objectives for older adults are limited to objectives on dementias, injury prevention, and kidney disease, but there are no objectives that reflect the physical and social determinants of healthy aging, such as frailty, sensory deficits, social connectedness (i.e., to address loneliness or social isolation), or aspects of livability, such as universal design elements that makes residences, commercial structures, sidewalks, and other parts of the built environment broadly accessible (see, for example, the AARP Livability Index [AARP, 2018]).

Well-being, health equity, and collaboration across multiple sectors represent some of the key aspects of the HP2030 Framework, yet they are insufficiently reflected in the draft objectives. This includes upstream macro-level social structural factors related to patterns of opportunity and risk within society, including employment rates, structural racism, residential segregation, wealth accumulation, and access to health care services, and the public policies that influence these patterns. In addition, there are few objectives that capture community or neighborhood-level factors for which there is strong evidence of a relationship to health

---

[7] See https://www.healthypeople.gov/2020/leading-health-indicators/2020-lhi-topics/Maternal-Infant-and-Child-Health (accessed July 16, 2019).

and availability of high-quality data, including data related to housing affordability and stability,[8] air quality, food availability, public safety, educational attainment, and poverty. In fact, objectives linked to four of the five key domains related to the social determinants of health from HP2020 are missing, including the domains of economic stability, education, neighborhood and built environment, and social and community context. The only domain that is well represented is that of clinical care. The shortage of objectives for the other four domains, including measures of community well-being, is a noteworthy and critical gap in the current iteration of draft objectives.

Several important analyses have emerged over the past two decades that have sought to quantify the relative contributions of various factors on health, such as the proportion of mortality attributable to smoking versus medical treatment versus education attainment. These include the work of McGinnis et al. (2002), the Booske et al. (2010) schema for weighting the different influences on health for the County Health Rankings model, and the more recent work from Kaplan and Milstein (2019). The pathways by which upstream social factors shape health and well-being are characterized by multiple interactions and a great deal of complexity (Braveman and Gottlieb, 2014); therefore, all available analyses have limitations, and the relative contributions of various factors surely do not add up to 100 percent (see Krieger, 2017). Given the modest contribution of medical care to health outcomes, and the robust evidence that factors ranging from income inequality, to adverse childhood experiences, to housing instability considerably influence population health, it is striking that the draft core objectives are largely oriented toward clinical measures/measures of health states. Although those measures are necessary, they are insufficient as a representation of the health and well-being of the nation or of communities.

Having reviewed the HP2020 evidence-based resources (and scoring system),[9] the committee noted, for example, that despite the evidence base for tenant-based rental assistance programs and despite the contemporary housing crisis faced by many American communities, with considerable implications for their health,[10] there is no reference to rental assistance

---

[8] See https://www.healthaffairs.org/do/10.1377/hpb20180313.396577/full (accessed July 16, 2019).

[9] See https://www.healthypeople.gov/2020/Implement/EBR-glossary#4-star (accessed July 2, 2019).

[10] See Taylor, 2018 (https://www.healthaffairs.org/do/10.1377/hpb20180313.396577/full, accessed July 2, 2019); and also the *Healthy People 2020* discussion about the quality of housing and implications for health.

among the HP2030 objectives.[11] There are many areas of robust evidence on social, physical, and environmental factors that shape health and well-being, but the objectives do not include a sufficient array to reflect such multisectoral contributions.

The objectives lack any mention of health equity (an HP2030 foundational principle) or addressing health disparities, there are no health equity measures, and some objectives give rise to questions about exacerbating certain types of inequities (to include ethnicity/race, gender, geographical, economic, and others as described in the health equity criterion for the HP2030 objectives). For example, because there is no objective related to life expectancy (especially surprising given the overall decline in life expectancy), there is also no focus on reducing the significant disparities in life expectancy by race in the United States. Similarly, reducing racial/ethnic and socioeconomic differences in leading causes of morbidity and mortality, such as cardiovascular disease, cancer, diabetes, and suicide, is a fundamental prerequisite for improving overall population health in the United States.

As another example, a family planning objective focuses on increasing "the proportion of females in need of publicly supported contraceptive services and supplies who receive those services and supplies" but misses the opportunity to measure males' use of public family planning, embodying the unfair expectation that women ought to manage contraception, placing a logistical and resource burden on females, thus leading to increased inequity. Additional objectives related to power and civic participation, such as measures of voter enfranchisement or voting registration are missing (Blakely et al., 2001; Chandra, 2019).

The committee has read the recommendations made by the SAC in its Report 7 (SAC, 2019b), which contains a review of the draft objectives, and believes that if the SAC's recommendations are implemented, they are likely to strengthen the final set of HP2030 objectives, providing a more well-rounded and HP2030 Framework-aligned complement of core objectives from which to select LHIs.

Finding 3: The committee finds that the *Healthy People 2030* draft objectives document includes too few objectives that allow for making important comparisons to other countries, including to peer nations in the Organisation for Economic Co-operation and Development.

---

[11] See https://www.healthypeople.gov/2020/tools-resources/evidence-based-resource/housing-tenant-based-rental-assistance-programs%E2%80%94-social (accessed July 2, 2019). See also newer evidence on supportive housing and health care cost savings at https://www.rand.org/pubs/research_reports/RR1694.html (accessed July 2, 2019).

This finding is referring not to rates of specific health outcomes, but rather, broader measures of population health such as life expectancy at birth, healthy life expectancy, or neonatal mortality. This could also include such measures as immunization coverage rates; social protection factors such as health insurance coverage, disability insurance, and parental leave; and well-being indicators such as civic engagement and trust in government, personal economic security, work–life balance, and subjective well-being.[12] Given the poor performance of the United States in global health rankings, noted in previous reports from the Institute of Medicine (IOM, 2012, 2013) and elsewhere (CIA, 2019; IHME, 2018), providing summary measures of population health and employing indicators used by peer nations could be helpful. A nation's health cannot be measured in a vacuum—international comparisons contribute an important aspect to ascertaining a nation's performance on key indicators. That is analogous to the state-to-state or county-to-county comparisons informed by such indicator efforts as America's Health Rankings and County Health Rankings, respectively.

ON OBJECTIVES FROM OTHER SECTORS IMPORTANT TO HEALTH AND WELL-BEING

Although *Healthy People 2030* emphasizes that well-being is produced not only by health sectors, but across all sectors of society, we note that only a small subset of the data sources for the HP2030 draft objectives reside outside the health domain. These include data from the Department of Agriculture, Department of Education, Department of Housing and Urban Development, and Department of Transportation. However, some departments remain underrepresented, and the objectives that draw on data from the aforementioned departments are small in number, narrow in scope, and not reflective of the full breadth of domains where moderate or robust evidence may be available to inform action. As noted above, the committee believes that the topic area on the social determinants of health is overly limited and more objectives are needed to provide adequate material for deriving some of the LHIs. Similar suggestions were made by the SAC in its Report 7 (SAC, 2019b).

A great deal has been written elsewhere about the fact that the macrosocial upstream factors that shape health outcomes, ranging from educational attainment to housing, reside in other sectors and are the responsibility of other government agencies, organizations, and disciplines (see, for example, NASEM, 2017). At the same time, however, communities

---

[12] See, for example, presentations given at the May 28, 2019, committee information-gathering meeting.

and states around the country are recognizing that the common good of all who reside in a community or state requires cross-sector dialogue and collaborative action. This is beginning to occur in many places. Some examples at different levels of government and from the private sector underscore that this is a moment of great opportunity for cross-sector collaboration including in the realm of metrics. The U.S. Surgeon General's initiative and forthcoming report on community health and economic prosperity acknowledges the linkages among employers, communities, health care organizations, and others.[13] The state of California has for nearly a decade had a Strategic Growth Council that includes a Health in All Policies Task Force.[14] Several federal government departments or agencies have set goals that could align with the Healthy People effort. For example, several federal departments and agencies list emergency preparedness and response activities in their strategic plans, such as the Department of Homeland Security, Department of the Interior, and the Small Business Administration.[15] In terms of the social determinants of health, the Department of Education, Department of Housing and Urban Development, and Department of the Treasury address issues such as educational attainment, sustainable homeownership, housing security, and safety in their strategic plans as well.[16] In considering health exposures and outcomes, the language in the strategic plans of the Department of Transportation and the Environmental Protection Agency aligns with HP2030 objectives related to protecting air quality and ensuring clean and safe water, and reducing the number of fatalities and serious injuries, respectively.

Another example of an area of alignment may be found in the Department of Education highlighting absenteeism as a key metric of educational success.[17] Research from the George W. Bush Presidential Center and the Brookings Institution,[18] among others, has explored the relationships among health, educational attainment, absenteeism, and other

---

[13] See https://www.hhs.gov/sites/default/files/community-health-and-economic-prosperity-infographic.pdf (accessed July 2, 2019).

[14] See http://sgc.ca.gov/programs/hiap (accessed July 2, 2019).

[15] Department of Homeland Security: https://www.dhs.gov/sites/default/files/publications/ST_Strategic_Plan_2015_508.pdf (accessed July 2, 2019); Department of the Interior: https://www.doi.gov/sites/doi.gov/files/uploads/fy2018-2022-strategic-plan.pdf (accessed July 2, 2019); Small Business Administration: https://www.sba.gov/sites/default/files/files/FINAL-2017-SBA-Disaster-Preparedness-Plan-signed.pdf (accessed July 2, 2019).

[16] See information gathered from a search of Performance.gov federal department or agency strategic plans and identification of items that appeared congruent with the HP2030 vision and mission.

[17] See https://www2.ed.gov/datastory/chronicabsenteeism.html (accessed June 27, 2019).

[18] See https://www.bushcenter.org/stateofourcities/spotlight/chronicabsenteeism (accessed July 2, 2019).

community factors. At the local level, other examples of cross-sector partnerships to improve health and well-being exist around the country. Richmond, California, has been a pioneer in adopting a health-in-all-policies approach in public–private collaboration involving the city and county;[19] the city of Appleton in Wisconsin has enacted a Health in All Policies ordinance; Fairfax County, Virginia, has a health-in-all-policies program and a health-in-all-policies manager that engages with other government agencies in the county; and Kent County, Michigan, has a Health in All Policies learning lab and toolkit.[20]

[19] See https://www.phi.org/uploads/files/Health_in_All_Policies-A_Guide_for_State_and_Local_Governments.pdf (accessed July 2, 2019).

[20] See https://www.appleton.org/home/showdocument?id=22076 (accessed July 2, 2019); https://www.fairfaxcounty.gov/livehealthy/sites/livehealthy/files/assets/documents/pdf/community-health-improvement-plan.pdf, pp. 3, 16 (accessed July 2, 2019); https://www.accesskent.com/Health/HiAP (accessed July 2, 2019).

4

Criteria for *Healthy People 2030* Leading Health Indicators

The Secretary's Advisory Committee on National Health Promotion and Disease Prevention Objectives for 2030 (SAC) has proposed a two-phase process for selecting Leading Health Indicators (LHIs) from the *Healthy People 2030* (HP2030) objectives (again, the objectives are currently available in draft form, with the final set expected in 2020). In phase 1 of the LHI selection process, all core objectives should be assessed across the following four criteria:

1. *Public health burden*—relative significance to the health and well-being of the nation;
2. *Magnitude of the health disparity* and the *degree to which health equity would be achieved* if the target were met;
3. The degree to which the objective is a *sentinel* or *bellwether*; and
4. *Actionability* of the objective.

In phase 2, the following four criteria are applied to the set of potential LHIs emerging from phase 1:

1. "The LHIs represent a *balanced portfolio* or cohesive set of indicators of health and well-being across the life span.
2. The LHIs are balanced between common, *upstream root causes* of poor health and well-being and measures of *high-priority health states*.
3. The LHIs are amenable to *policy, environmental, and systems* interventions at the local, state, tribal, and national levels.

4. The LHIs are *understandable* and will *resonate* with diverse stakeholders to drive action" (SAC, 2018a, pp. 3, 4).

The committee has reviewed the criteria in the two-phase process for selection of the LHIs. The SAC's description of the phases and criteria, and the rationale for each, are provided in the SAC's report on the LHIs (see Appendix D). As noted above, the LHIs are defined by the SAC as a "selected set of measures of determinants and sentinel indicators of current and potential changes in population health and well-being" and "drawn from Healthy People objectives to communicate the highest-priority health issues." Highest-priority health issues, the National Academies of Sciences, Engineering, and Medicine committee adds, would include not only those that characterize the health of the country, but also, the health of communities.

The committee agrees with the phase 1 and phase 2 criteria for the LHI selection—they cover all essential characteristics of individual LHIs and a well-constructed set of LHIs, and they are also consistent with previously described criteria (e.g., previous reports from the National Academies that addressed the criteria for selecting a small set of indicators). The committee notes that the main goal of phase 1 is to ensure that the LHIs meet certain specific criteria, such as public health burden, that demonstrate their importance to the nation's health and well-being. The main goal of phase 2 appears to be a diagnostic check on phase 1 to ensure that the selected LHIs comport with the ideas identified in phase 0 (the proposed additional phase discussed below).

The committee has a few observations to share about the LHI criteria. Regarding the phase 1 criteria, "The magnitude of the health disparity and the degree to which health equity would be achieved if the target were met" seems to be a fairly aspirational criterion, because the data needed for this kind of analysis are often not available. The second criterion in phase 2—balancing upstream root causes with high-priority health states—may need to be applied earlier, perhaps as part of phase 1, given the importance of having a set of LHIs that addresses both upstream root causes and high-priority health states. The third criterion in phase 2, that "LHIs are amenable to policy, environmental, and systems interventions at the local, state, tribal, and national levels," a criterion to be applied to the full complement of the LHIs, may need to be revised to replace the *and* in "local, state, tribal, and national levels" with an *or*, as it does not seem realistic to expect that each LHI would be amenable to interventions of all types at every level.

As noted, the draft core objectives from which the LHIs are to be derived are currently characterized by the limitations described above—the collection of draft objectives offers both too much and too little for identifying the LHIs that are aligned with the HP2030 Framework. It is easy to get lost in the minutiae of myriad objectives, but the HP2030 Framework offers a coherent vision and pathway, one that also seems well aligned with the frameworks for national or local indicators showcased at the National Academies committee's May 28, 2019, information-gathering meeting (NASEM, 2019). The HP2030 Framework developed by the SAC appears designed to balance the need for continuity with the past with the need to evolve to meet emerging and future opportunities and challenges. However, given that the LHI selection criteria begin by calling for assessing "all core objectives," having objectives that are minimally aligned with the HP2030 Framework may lead to an inadequate, subjective, and ineffective process of identifying indicators to serve the field in the future. Providing a more well-rounded collection of objectives that show the "big picture" articulated by the Framework will be essential to ensuring that meaningful and useful LHIs can be selected.

Finding 4: The committee finds that if the existing criteria for Leading Health Indicator (LHI) selection were applied to the existing *Healthy People 2030* draft objectives, the resulting LHI set would not be aligned with the *Healthy People 2030* Framework—it would not tell a coherent story about the nation's (or communities') health, well-being, and the state of health equity.

Therefore:

Recommendation 1: The committee recommends that the Department of Health and Human Services and the Federal Interagency Workgroup add to the *Healthy People 2030* objectives topics or implement a structural reorganization (with additional topics) that will yield more core objectives that reflect the *Healthy People 2030* Framework and could lead to better Leading Health Indicators. Cross-cutting topics (i.e., topics that refer to or link with multiple health states, life stages, systems, and all dimensions of health) should include health equity; the social, physical, and economic determinants of health; shared responsibility and multiple sectors; and all levels of government.

Inspired by the SAC's efforts in framing the *Healthy People 2030* initiative, the committee also recommends the following:

Recommendation 2: The committee recommends a three-phase process should be used for Leading Health Indicator (LHI) selection from the *Healthy People 2030* objectives. A new phase would

precede the existing two, and it would apply the *Healthy People 2030* Framework (especially the vision, mission, foundational principles, and overarching goals) in consideration of additional objectives and in selecting LHIs.

The term *phases* implies a chronological sequence; however, the committee notes that the term *filter* may more accurately describe the manner in which criteria would likely be applied, and also includes a recognition that some of the criteria from phase 1 and phase 2 may in fact be applied concurrently. The main goal of adding a new phase (or filter) to the LHI selection process, let us call it phase 0, would be to ensure that the major concepts of the HP2030 Framework are represented in the LHIs as a collective set.

The existing objectives could remain under consideration as LHIs in accordance with the guidance already provided by the SAC in Report 7, but additional selection criteria are needed to determine which objectives can be the LHIs. The committee believes that the three-phase process recommended is needed to help "see the forest for the trees" among all the currently proposed objectives/indicators, and to operationalize the vision, mission, foundational principles, and goals of HP2030 in "filtering" the vast range of indicators represented in the collection of HP2030 draft core objectives.

5

Conclusion

The committee is grateful for the opportunity to provide input about the criteria for selecting Leading Health Indicators (LHIs), and looks forward to offering additional input in our second report in the form of recommendations for core objectives and the LHIs themselves. The committee has noted that the Secretary's Advisory Committee on National Health Promotion and Disease Prevention Objectives for 2030 (SAC) and the Department of Health and Human Services are developing communication plans with attention to a wide range of stakeholders and implementing partners for *Healthy People 2030* (SAC, 2018c). The committee commends the broad-based approach reflected in the work of the SAC, including the development of supplemental briefs that shed light on the SAC's thinking about the foundational principles in the *Healthy People 2030* (HP2030) Framework. The committee affirms the importance of having LHIs that address that broad approach.

The LHI criteria include that when viewed as a group, LHIs are "balanced between common, upstream root causes of health and well-being and measures of high-priority health states" and are "understandable and will resonate with diverse stakeholders to drive action." The latter criterion calls for dissemination and communication, the importance of which is underscored by the fact many people may equate health with medical care and may be unfamiliar with the contributions to health and well-being of nonclinical factors such as education and social cohesion (Ortiz and Johannes, 2018; Robert and Booske, 2011). Although the understanding among the experts of what creates health and well-being is changing rapidly, approximately one-third of Americans recognize that their surroundings influence their health (Carman et al., 2019). *Healthy People 2030* offers an exceptional opportunity toward creating a shared understanding of what is needed, beyond medical care and its complexity, to build the conditions for health and well-being, and thus, toward influencing a balanced portfolio of investments in what can make the nation and its communities healthier, more vibrant, and more prosperous. Those approaches and investments are needed to address both behaviors and individual decision making, as well as sociodemographics—the "upstream" and ecological factors that shape individual decisions and trajectories (Lantz et al., 2010).

Many Americans are uninformed about inequity and its structural and historic causes (Pew, 2019). The LHIs offer an opportunity to highlight the state of upstream social structural factors that drive social disparities in health and well-being, and show that racial health inequities impose a broader cost on society (LaVeist et al., 2011). U.S. communities and states are also facing several macroeconomic and environmental threats that may present serious challenges to the work of promoting health and well-being. The LHIs provide an important opportunity to put in place some key tracking mechanisms that highlight the relationships among health and well-being and such factors as wealth inequality, mass incarceration, and unaffordable housing.

Appendix A

References

AARP. 2018. *AARP Livability Index: Transforming communities for all ages*. https://www.aarp.org/content/dam/aarp/ppi/2018/06/livability-index-transforming-communities-for-all-ages.pdf (accessed July 24, 2019).

Azar, A. 2018. Charter. In *Secretary's Advisory Committee on National Health Promotion and Disease Prevention Objectives for 2030*. Washington, DC: Department of Health and Human Services.

Blakely, T. A., B. P. Kennedy, and I. Kawachi. 2001. Socioeconomic inequality in voting participation and self-rated health. *American Journal of Public Health* 91(1):99–104. doi: 10.2105/ajph.91.1.99.

Booske, B. C., J. K. Athens, D. A. Kindig, H. Park, and P. L. Remington. 2010. *County Health Rankings working paper: Different perspectives for assigning weights to determinants of health.* Madison, WI: University of Wisconsin–Madison, Population Health Institute.

Braveman, P. 2014. What are health disparities and health equity? We need to be clear. *Public Health Report* 129(Suppl 2):5–8. doi: 10.1177/00333549141291S203.

Braveman, P., and L. Gottlieb. 2014. The social determinants of health: It's time to consider the causes of the causes. *Public Health Reports* 129(Suppl 2):19–31.

Chandra, A. 2019. *Presentation to the Committee on the Selection of Leading Health Indicators for* Healthy People 2030. http://www.nationalacademies.org/hmd/~/media/Files/Activity%20Files/PublicHealth/HealthyPeople2030/May%2028%20presentations/Session%202-1%20Chandra.pdf (accessed June 21, 2019).

CIA (Central Intelligence Agency). 2019. *The World Factbook. Country Comparison: Life expectancy at birth.* https://www.cia.gov/library/publications/the-world-factbook/rankorder/2102rank.html (accessed July 24, 2019).

HHS (Department of Health and Human Services). 2018. *Secretary's Advisory Committee on National Health Promotion and Disease Prevention Objectives for 2030: 9th Meeting Summary, May 14, 2018.* https://www.healthypeople.gov/2020/About-Healthy-People/Development-Healthy-People-2030/Committee-Meetings (accessed July 25, 2019).

HHS. 2019a. *Healthy People [2020] Leading Health Indicators development and framework.* https://www.healthypeople.gov/2020/leading-health-indicators/Leading-Health-Indicators-Development-and-Framework (accessed June 20, 2019).

HHS. 2019b. *Proposed objectives for inclusion in* Healthy People 2030. https://www.healthypeople.gov/sites/default/files/ObjectivesPublicComment508_1.17.19.pdf (accessed June 20, 2019).

HHS. n.d. *Evidence-based resources frequently asked questions (FAQs).* https://www.healthypeople.gov/2020/Implement/EBR-glossary#selection-criteria (accessed July 24, 2019).

IHME (Institute for Health Metrics and Evaluation). 2018. United States profile. Seattle, WA: Institute for Health Metrics and Evaluation, University of Washington, 2018. http://www.healthdata.org/united-states (accessed July 23, 2019).

IOM (Institute of Medicine). 1999. *Leading health indicators for* Healthy People 2010. Washington, DC: National Academy Press.

IOM. 2011. *Leading health indicators for* Healthy People 2020. Washington, DC: The National Academies Press.

IOM. 2012. *For the public's health: Investing in a healthier future.* Washington, DC: The National Academies Press.

IOM. 2013. *Toward quality measures for population health and the Leading Health Indicators.* Washington, DC: The National Academies Press.

IOM. 2015. *Vital signs: Core metrics for health and health care progress.* Washington, DC: The National Academies Press.

Kaplan, R. M., and A. Milstein. 2019. Contributions of health care to longevity: A review of 4 estimation methods. *Annals of Family Medicine* 17:267–272. doi: 10.1370/afm.2362.

Krieger, N. 2017. Health equity and the fallacy of treating causes of population health as if they sum to 100%. *American Journal of Public Health* 107(4):541–549.

Lantz, P. M., E. Golberstein, J. S. House, and J. Morenoff. 2010. Social and behavioral risk factors for mortality in a national 19-year prospective study of U.S. adults. *Social Science & Medicine* 70:1558–1566.

LaVeist, T. A., D. Gaskin, and P. Richard. 2011. Estimating the economic burden of racial health inequalities in the United States. *International Journal of Health Sciences* 41(2):231–238.

McGinnis, J. M., P. Williams-Russo, and J. Knickman. 2002. The case for more active policy attention to health promotion. *Health Affairs* 21(20):78–93.

NASEM (National Academies of Sciences, Engineering, and Medicine). 2017. *Communities in action: Pathways to health equity.* Washington, DC: The National Academies Press.

NASEM. 2019. *Meeting 3: Committee on Informing the Selection of Leading Health Indicators for Healthy People 2030.* Washington, DC. http://nationalacademies.org/hmd/Activities/PublicHealth/LeadingHealthIndicatorsForHealthyPeople2030/2019-MAY-28.aspx (accessed July 2, 2019).

NCHS (National Center for Health Statistics). 2010. Healthy People 2010 *final review: Leading Health Indicators.* https://www.cdc.gov/nchs/data/hpdata2010/hp2010_final_review_leading_health_indicators.pdf (accessed May 21, 2019).

Ortiz, S. E., and B. L. Johannes. 2018. Building the case for housing policy: Understanding public beliefs about housing affordability as a key social determinant of health. *SSM–Population Health* 6:63–71. doi: 10.1016/j.ssmph.2018.08.008.

Robert, S. A., and B. C. Booske. 2011. US opinions on health determinants and social policy as health policy. *American Journal of Public Health* 101(9):1655–1663. doi: 10.2105/AJPH.2011.300217.

SAC (Secretary's Advisory Committee on National Health Promotion and Disease Prevention Objectives for 2020). 2010. *Evidence-based clinical and public health: Generating and applying the evidence.* https://www.healthypeople.gov/sites/default/files/EvidenceBasedClinicalPH2010.pdf (accessed July 24, 2019).

SAC (Secretary's Advisory Committee on National Health Promotion and Disease Prevention Objectives for 2030). 2018a. *Recommendations for the* Healthy People 2030 *Leading Health Indicators*. Washington, DC: Department of Health and Human Services.

SAC. 2018b. *Recommendations for developing objectives, setting priorities, identifying data needs, and involving stakeholders for* Healthy People 2030. Report 2. Washington, DC: Department of Health and Human Services.

SAC. 2018c. *Stakeholder engagement and communication for* Healthy People 2030. Report 5. Washington, DC: Department of Health and Human Services.

SAC. 2019a. *Issue briefs to inform development and implementation of* Healthy People 2030. https://www.healthypeople.gov/sites/default/files/Committee-LHI-Report-to-Secretary_1.pdf (accessed July 18, 2019).

SAC. 2019b. *Assessment and recommendations for proposed objectives for* Healthy People 2030. Report 7. Washington, DC: Department of Health and Human Services.

Taylor, L. 2018. Housing and health: An overview of the literature. *Health Affairs Health Policy Brief*, June 7, 2018. doi: 10.1377/hpb20180313.396577.

WHO (World Health Organization). 2014. *Constitution of the World Health Organization*. http://apps.who.int/gb/bd/PDF/bd48/basic-documents-48th-edition-en.pdf#page=7 (accessed June 20, 2019).

Appendix B

Meeting Agendas

MEETING 1: FEBRUARY 27, 2019

2:00 pm Welcome and Introductions
George Isham, HealthPartners Institute (Committee Chair)

2:10 pm Giving of the Charge and Context
Carter Blakey, Office of Disease Prevention and Health Promotion, Office of the Assistant Secretary for Health, Department of Health and Human Services (HHS)

2:45 pm Q&A

3:00 pm Adjourn

MEETING 2: APRIL 19, 2019

12:00 pm Welcome and Introductions
George Isham, HealthPartners Institute (Committee Chair)

12:10 pm Update About the *Healthy People 2030* Initiative
Don Wright, Deputy Assistant Secretary for Health, Director, Office of Disease Prevention and Health Promotion, HHS

12:20 pm Remarks About the Work of the Secretary's Advisory Committee on National Health Promotion and Disease Prevention Objectives for 2030
Dushanka Kleinman, Professor and Principal Associate Dean for Research, University of Maryland School of Public Health, University of Maryland (HHS Secretary's Advisory Committee[1] Co-Chair)
Nico Pronk, President, HealthPartners Institute (HHS Secretary's Advisory Committee Co-Chair)

12:50 pm Questions from the National Academies Committee

1:20 pm Break

1:35 pm Remarks About the Work of the Subcommittee on Leading Health Indicators
Therese Richmond, Andrea B. Laporte Professor of Nursing; Associate Dean for Research & Innovation, School of Nursing, University of Pennsylvania (Chair, Subcommittee on Leading Health Indicators)

2:05 pm Questions from the National Academies Committee

2:35 pm Public Comment (time permitting)

3:00 pm Adjourn

MEETING 3: MAY 28, 2019

9:00 am Welcome and Introductions
George Isham, HealthPartners Institute (Committee Chair)

9:15 am Presentation from the Deputy Assistant Secretary of Health
Don Wright, HHS

[1] Secretary's Advisory Committee on National Health Promotion and Disease Prevention Objectives for 2030.

9:30 am	Perspectives on the Purpose and Use of Leading Health Indicators (LHIs) (or a Small High-Level Set of Indicators for the Nation More Broadly) with Both National and Community Needs in Mind Moderator: Terry Richmond, University of Pennsylvania Anita Chandra, RAND Bobby Milstein, ReThink Health Soma Stout, Institute for Healthcare Improvement and 100 Million Healthier Lives Carley Riley, Cincinnati Children's and 100 Million Healthier Lives
10:30 am	Break
10:45 am	Q&A Moderator: George Isham
11:10 am	Data Sources for Objectives and the LHIs Moderator: Ed Sondik, formerly National Center for Health Statistics Ali Mokdad, Institute for Health Metrics and Evaluation Amy O'Hara, Massive Data Institute, McCourt School of Public Policy, Georgetown University
11:55 am	Q&A Moderator: George Isham
12:15 pm	Lunch
1:15 pm	Harmonizing with Other National Metrics Sets Moderator: Dushanka Kleinman, University of Maryland Tom Eckstein, Arundel Metrics Kristen Lewis, Social Science Research Council Marjory Givens, University of Wisconsin–Madison (via Zoom)
2:15 pm	Q&A Moderator: George Isham
2:40 pm	Break

2:55 pm	Measuring Health Equity—Insights for the LHIs
	Moderator: Nico Pronk, HealthPartners Institute
	    Brian Smedley, National Collaborative for Health Equity
	    Steven Woolf, Virginia Commonwealth University (absent)
	    Sarah Treuhaft, Policy Link (via Zoom)

3:40 pm	Q&A Moderator: George Isham
4:00 pm	Public Comment (time permitting)
4:15 pm	Adjourn

Appendix C

Committee Member Biosketches[1]

George J. Isham, M.D., M.S. (*Chair*), is currently a Senior Fellow at the HealthPartners Institute in Minneapolis, Minnesota. His areas of interest include understanding how health is created in populations and how to improve health and health care quality and financing. He is formerly a Senior Advisor (2012–2017) and Medical Director and Chief Health Officer (1993–2012) at HealthPartners. He is also currently a Senior Advisor to the Alliance of Community Health Plans and a member of the advisory board for the Center for Health Economics and Policy at FTI Consulting. Dr. Isham is an elected member of the National Academy of Medicine and was designated as a National Associate of the Institute of Medicine in 2003 in recognition of his contribution to its work. He has chaired the National Academies' Roundtable on Population Health Improvement and the Roundtable on Health Literacy; chaired, served, and reviewed for a number of consensus study reports; and participated in a number of National Academies workshops. Dr. Isham has been active in health policy, serving as a former member of the Centers for Disease Control and Prevention's (CDC's) Task Force on Community Preventive Services, as a member of the Agency for Healthcare Research and Quality's U.S. Preventive Services Task Force, and was a founding Co-Chair of the National Committee for Quality Assurance's committee on performance measurement as well as a founding Co-Chair of the National Quality Forum's Measurement Application Partnership. He is a founding member of the

---

[1] The members of the committee serve on the committee as individuals rather than as representatives of their respective organizations.

advisory board for the National Guideline Clearinghouse and has served on the Advisory Committee to the Director of CDC.

Dr. Isham earned his bachelor of arts degree in zoology and master of science in preventive medicine/administrative medicine from the University of Wisconsin–Madison, and his doctor of medicine from the University of Illinois in Chicago. He completed his internship and residency in internal medicine at the University of Wisconsin Hospital and Clinics in Madison, Wisconsin. Dr. Isham has clinical experience as a general medical officer in the U.S. Navy, in the general practice of internal medicine at the Freeport Clinic in Freeport, Illinois, and as a Clinical Assistant Professor of Medicine at the University of Wisconsin Hospitals and Clinics in Madison, Wisconsin.

Ebony Boulware, M.D., M.P.H., is a Professor of Medicine, Chief of the Division of General Internal Medicine in the Department of Medicine, Vice Dean for Translational Science, and Associate Vice Chancellor for Translational Research in the School of Medicine at Duke University. She received an A.B. from Vassar College, an M.D. from Duke University, and an M.P.H. from the Johns Hopkins Bloomberg School of Public Health. Dr. Boulware is a General Internist and a Clinical Epidemiologist. She attended medical school at Duke University, completed medical training as a resident and chief resident at the University of Maryland, and she completed a research fellowship at the Johns Hopkins University School of Medicine. She became a faculty member in the Johns Hopkins University School of Medicine and Bloomberg School of Public Health in 2002, where she achieved the academic rank of Full Professor. In 2013, she was appointed Chief of the Division of General Internal Medicine in the Department of Medicine at Duke University. In 2015, she was appointed the inaugural Director of the Duke Clinical and Translational Science Institute, and she is the contact Principal Investigator for the Duke Clinical and Translational Science Award for Duke University. Dr. Boulware has devoted her scholarly career to studying mechanisms to improve the quality and equity of health care and health outcomes for patients and populations with chronic diseases such as chronic kidney disease and hypertension. As part of her work, she investigates the influence of attitudinal, social, and environmental contexts on health and health outcomes. She has maintained an active research portfolio throughout her career, funded by the National Institutes of Health, the Patient-Centered Outcomes Research Institute, the Health Resources and Services Administration, the Agency for Healthcare Research and Quality, and several foundations. She has published more than 120 manuscripts, and she has mentored numerous students, fellows, and faculty members in clinical research. Dr. Boulware frequently engages community members, patients, their family members, and other stakeholders to develop and implement relevant and sustainable interventions to improve health.

Gilbert Gee, Ph.D., is a Professor in the Department of Community Health Sciences at the UCLA Fielding School of Public Health at the University of California, Los Angeles. He received his bachelor's degree in neuroscience from Oberlin College, his doctorate in Health Policy and Management from the Johns Hopkins University, and postdoctoral training in sociology from Indiana University. His research focuses on the social determinants of health inequities of racial, ethnic, and immigrant minority populations using a multilevel and life course perspective. A primary line of his research focuses on conceptualizing and measuring racial discrimination, and in understanding how discrimination may be related to illness. He has also published more broadly on the topics of stress, neighborhoods, environmental exposures, occupational health, and on Asian American populations. Current projects include the study of discrimination; racial identity and obesity among emigrants from the Philippines; the relationship between student loans and illness; and toxic exposures among Asian American participants in a National Health and Nutrition Examination Survey. His research has been honored with a group Merit Award from the National Institutes of Health for the development of multicultural measures of discrimination for health surveys. In addition, he received two Scientific and Technical Achievement Awards from the Environmental Protection Agency for development of the Stress-Exposure-Disease Framework.

Marthe R. Gold, M.D., M.P.H., is a Senior Scholar at The New York Academy of Medicine, and the Logan Professor Emeritus in the Department of Community Health and Social Medicine at the City University of New York Medical School. A graduate of the Tufts University School of Medicine and the Columbia School of Public Health, her clinical training is in family medicine. Dr. Gold has been a Primary Care Provider in urban and rural underserved settings. She served as Senior Policy Adviser in the Office of the Assistant Secretary for Health in the Department of Health and Human Services from 1990 to 1996 where her focus was on financing of clinical preventive services, the economics and outcomes of public health programs, and health care reform. She directed the work of the Panel on Cost-Effectiveness in Health and Medicine, an expert panel whose report remains an influential guide to cost-effectiveness methodology for academic and policy uses. Her current work focuses on patient, public, and decision maker views on using economic and comparative effectiveness information to inform health policy. A member of the National Academy of Medicine, Dr. Gold served as Chair of its

Committee on Public Health Strategies to Improve Health (reports published 2010–2012) and has been a member of the Roundtable on Population Health Improvement since its inception.

Sheri Johnson, Ph.D., is the Director of the Population Health Institute (PHI) at the University of Wisconsin–Madison, Visiting Associate Professor, and Acting Director, County Health Rankings & Roadmaps, and the Robert Wood Johnson Foundation Culture of Health Prize. For more than 25 years Dr. Johnson has dedicated her career to partnering with children, families, community organizations, and systems to advance health and well-being. Awed by the resilience of individuals and communities, she is motivated to remove unfair obstacles and conditions that create and perpetuate health inequities. Dr. Johnson completed her undergraduate studies at Brown University, earned an M.A. and a Ph.D. in clinical psychology at Boston University, and served as a Clinical Fellow in psychology at Harvard Medical School. She was previously the Director of Behavioral Health at Milwaukee Health Services, Inc., a federally qualified health center, and served as the Administrator and State Health Officer for the Wisconsin Division of Public Health. Immediately prior to joining the PHI, she was Associate Professor of Pediatrics at the Medical College of Wisconsin Center for Advancement of Underserved Children where she collaborated with diverse stakeholders to address a broad range of real-world problems.

Paula Lantz, Ph.D., is the Associate Dean for academic affairs and a Professor of public policy at the Ford School. She also holds an appointment as Professor of health management and policy in the School of Public Health. Dr. Lantz, a social demographer, studies the role of public policy in improving population health. She currently directs the University of Michigan Policies for Action Research Hub, funded by the Robert Wood Johnson Foundation, which is engaged in a number of research projects investigating public policy approaches to reducing social inequities in health. Dr. Lantz is leading a project regarding the potential for and challenges associated with using social impact bonds to fund public–private partnerships aimed at improving population health. An elected member of the National Academy of Social Insurance and the National Academy of Medicine, Dr. Lantz received an M.A. in sociology from Washington University in St. Louis, and an M.S. in epidemiology and a Ph.D. in sociology from the University of Wisconsin.

Darcy Phelan-Emrick, Dr.P.H., M.H.S., has served as the Chief Epidemiologist at the Baltimore City Health Department since 2015. She leads the Health Department's efforts to develop and track public health objectives and goals. Dr. Phelan-Emrick has been a full-time faculty member in the Department of Epidemiology at the Johns Hopkins University Bloomberg School of Public Health since 2009, and she holds a joint appointment in the Department of Health, Behavior and Society. She has held prior positions in the New York City Department of Health and Mental Hygiene, The New York Academy of Medicine, and The Rockefeller University. Dr. Phelan-Emrick received her Dr.P.H. in 2009 and M.H.S. in 2005, both in epidemiology, from the Johns Hopkins Bloomberg School of Public Health.

Jonathan S. Skinner, Ph.D., is a health economist with experience leading several research projects funded by the National Institute on Aging. These are large-scale interdisciplinary collaborations at Dartmouth College and involving partner institutions, drawing on Dartmouth's comprehensive Medicare and Medicaid data sets. Dr. Skinner's ongoing research focuses on studying the contribution of "high-tech" health care to cost growth, the diffusion of various types of medical innovations (beneficial and less so), how provider networks affect technology diffusion, and measuring efficiency in health care. A member of the National Academy of Medicine, Dr. Skinner is also a Research Associate and a Director of the Aging Program at the National Bureau of Economic Research. He has taught in Dartmouth's Department of Economics since 1995, where he serves as the James O. Freedman Presidential Professor.

Appendix D

Criteria for Selecting a Set of Leading Health Indicators[1]

Healthy People 2030 comprises three types of objectives—core, developmental, and research. The Leading Health Indicators (LHIs) for *Healthy People 2030* will be drawn from the core objectives because core objectives are defined as having valid, reliable, and timely data sources, as well as evidence-based interventions through which their targets can be met. The Committee proposes a set of criteria for selecting *Healthy People 2030* LHIs that are informed by the *Healthy People 2030* Framework, including the vision, mission, foundational principles, overarching goals, and plan of action.

PHASE 1

All core objectives should be assessed across the following four criteria:

1. *Public health burden*—relative significance to the health and well-being of the nation;
2. *Magnitude of the health disparity* and the *degree to which health equity would be achieved* if the target were met;
3. The degree to which the objective is a *sentinel* or *bellwether*; and
4. *Actionability* of the objective.

[1] SOURCE: The Secretary's Advisory Committee report *Recommendations for the Leading Health Indicators*.

Rationale

In phase 1, four criteria are applied to the core objectives. The first criterion, *public health burden*, is classically indicated by important metrics such as excess morbidity and mortality. Conversely, however, indicators may at first glance be viewed as having low public health burden (e.g., low levels of selected infectious diseases) owing to current practice (e.g., vaccinations). For this reason, public health burden must also be assessed by whether it would be significant if current practice were not continued. Public health burden directly supports the mission of *Healthy People 2030*, which is to "promote, strengthen, and evaluate the nation's efforts to improve the health and well-being of all people."

The second criterion focuses on the *magnitude of the health disparity and the degree to which health equity would be achieved if the LHI target were met*. It directly supports the overarching goal to "eliminate health disparities, achieve health equity, and attain health literacy to improve the health and well-being of all."

The third criterion emphasizes the role of the LHIs in serving as a *sentinel* and *bellwether* for the state of the nation's health and as a warning or harbinger of threats. This criterion supports the *Healthy People 2030* plan of action to "provide data that can drive targeted actions to address regions and populations with poor health or at high risk for poor health in the future."

Actionability, the final criterion, is multifaceted. It takes into account the state of available and actionable evidence, and the ability to improve health and well-being at a cost that is considered a good value. Actionability is informed by the foundational principle that "promoting and achieving the nation's health and well-being is a shared responsibility that is distributed across the national, state, tribal, and community levels, including the public, private, and not-for-profit sectors," and the plan of action to develop and make available "affordable means of health promotion, disease prevention, and treatment."

Description of Application

Phase 1 is a focused assessment that applies a set of four criteria to each core objective in *Healthy People 2030*. A quantitative approach helps identify the initial set of potential LHI candidates. All core objectives would be assessed according to each criterion on a scale of 1 (not important) to 10 (very important). A cumulative score would be calculated across the four criteria, ranging from 4 (least important) to 40 (most important). Those core objectives with the highest ranked scores would be considered as candidates for the pool of possible LHIs for *Healthy People 2030*.

PHASE 2

The pool of possible LHIs that emerges from phase 1 would then be subjected to an additional set of criteria before the final LHIs for *Healthy People 2030* are selected. The phase 2 criteria should be applied with the important assumption that the LHIs are to be viewed as a group. Individuals who apply these criteria to select the LHIs should assure the following:

- The LHIs represent a balanced portfolio or cohesive set of indicators of health and well-being across the life span.
- The LHIs are balanced between common, upstream root causes of poor health and well-being and measures of high-priority health states.
- The LHIs are amenable to policy, environmental, and systems interventions at the local, state, tribal, and national levels.
- The LHIs are understandable and will resonate with diverse stakeholders to drive action.

Rationale

Considerations for phase 2 reinforce the foundational principles upon which *Healthy People 2030* is based. They also reflect the *Healthy People 2030* vision—"a society in which all people can achieve their full potential for health and well-being across the life span"—with the intent of attaining lives free of preventable disease, disability, injury, and premature death. Achievement of balance between upstream root causes and measures of high-priority health states in the final set of the LHIs can be guided by the foundational principle that "healthy physical, social, and economic environments strengthen the potential to achieve health and well-being." The final two criteria in phase 2 emphasize the importance that the LHIs as a set resonate with diverse stakeholders who must take action. This notion is specified in the foundational principle "promoting and achieving the nation's health and well-being is a shared responsibility that is distributed across the national, state, tribal, and community levels, including the public, private, and not-for-profit sectors," and the centrality of *Healthy People 2030* as "a component of decision making and policy formulation across all sectors."

Description of Application

Unlike the core objectives, the LHIs do not exist in isolation from one another. Therefore, an additional assessment of the LHIs as a group is warranted. In this second phase, those who apply the additional criteria listed above would then evaluate the proposed set of the LHIs as a whole. As various sets of potential LHIs are constructed during this phase, it is likely and indeed recommended that iterative movement between phase 1 and phase 2 take place until the final set of the LHIs is selected. For example, it is possible that what emerges from the initial phase 1 process may not adequately balance the upstream root causes of poor health and well-being and measures of high-priority health states. It is also possible that the set would not resonate sufficiently across stakeholders to drive action.

Appendix E

Healthy People 2030 Framework[1]

HISTORY OF THE HEALTHY PEOPLE INITIATIVE

Healthy People is a national effort that sets goals and objectives to improve the health and well-being of people in the United States. *Healthy People 2030* is the fifth edition of Healthy People. It aims at new challenges and builds on lessons learned from its first four decades. The initiative began in 1979, when Surgeon General Julius Richmond issued a landmark report titled *Healthy People: The Surgeon General's Report on Health Promotion and Disease Prevention*. This report focused on reducing preventable death and injury. It included ambitious, quantifiable objectives to achieve national health promotion and disease prevention goals for the United States within a 10-year period (by 1990). The report was followed in later decades by the release of updated, 10-year Healthy People goals and objectives (*Healthy People 2000*, *Healthy People 2010*, and *Healthy People 2020*).

WHAT HEALTHY PEOPLE CONTRIBUTES

Healthy People helps users to access data on changes in the health status of the U.S. population; these data also inform each new decade's goals and objectives. Communities across the United States may adopt Healthy People goals and objectives. Communities, which may be as small as neighborhoods or large as municipalities, may alter the goals

[1] Prepared by the Secretary's Advisory Committee on National Health Promotion and Disease Prevention Objectives for 2030.

and objectives to meet their own needs and use them to set priorities for their region and population groups. Healthy People priorities are those aspects of health that are the most critical to overall health and well-being and can be improved using our available knowledge.

Since the Healthy People initiative was first launched, the United States has made significant progress. Achievements include reducing major causes of death such as heart disease and cancer; reducing infant and maternal mortality; reducing risk factors like tobacco smoking, hypertension, and elevated cholesterol; and increasing childhood vaccinations. During these decades, the importance of collaborating across agencies at the national, state, local, and tribal levels, and with the private and public health sectors, has been demonstrated.

A key lesson is that a widely accessible plan containing achievable goals and objectives can guide the action of individuals, communities, and stakeholders to improve health. To achieve the health and well-being of all people, it is essential to involve, as active partners, diverse stakeholders from across the public, private, and not-for-profit sectors. It is important to monitor progress on Healthy People goals and objectives, and to share high-quality data and feedback on progress with stakeholders and the public. In addition, we have learned that significant changes (e.g., reduced rates of smoking) may be difficult, but they are achievable through persistent effort.

Although much progress has been made, the United States lags behind other developed countries (such as other members of the Organisation for Economic Co-operation and Development) on key measures of health and well-being, including life expectancy, infant mortality, and obesity, despite spending the highest percentage of its gross domestic product on health. A challenge for *Healthy People 2030* is to guide the United States in achieving our population's full potential for health and well-being so we are second to none among developed countries.

VISION

A society in which all people can achieve their full potential for health and well-being across the life span.

MISSION

To promote, strengthen, and evaluate the nation's efforts to improve the health and well-being of all people.

FOUNDATIONAL PRINCIPLES

Foundational principles explain the thinking that guides decisions about *Healthy People 2030.*

1. Health and well-being of all people and communities are essential to a thriving, equitable society.
2. Promoting health and well-being and preventing disease are linked efforts that encompass physical, mental, and social health dimensions.
3. Investing to achieve the full potential for health and well-being for all provides valuable benefits to society.
4. Achieving health and well-being requires eliminating health disparities, achieving health equity, and attaining health literacy.
5. Healthy physical, social, and economic environments strengthen the potential to achieve health and well-being.
6. Promoting and achieving the nation's health and well-being is a shared responsibility that is distributed across the national, state, tribal, and community levels, including the public, private, and not-for-profit sectors.
7. Working to attain the full potential for health and well-being of the population is a component of decision making and policy formulation across all sectors.

OVERARCHING GOALS

1. Attain healthy, thriving lives and well-being, free of preventable disease, disability, injury, and premature death.
2. Eliminate health disparities, achieve health equity, and attain health literacy to improve the health and well-being of all.
3. Create social, physical, and economic environments that promote attaining full potential for health and well-being for all.
4. Promote healthy development, healthy behaviors, and well-being across all life stages.
5. Engage leadership, key constituents, and the public across multiple sectors to take action and design policies that improve the health and well-being of all.

PLAN OF ACTION

1. Set national goals and measurable objectives to guide evidence-based policies, programs, and other actions to improve health and well-being.

2. Provide data that are accurate, timely, accessible, and can drive targeted actions to address regions and populations with poor health or at high risk for poor health in the future.
3. Foster improvement through public and private efforts to improve health and well-being for people of all ages and the communities in which they live.
4. Provide tools for the public, programs, policy makers, and others to evaluate progress toward improving health and well-being.
5. Share and support the implementation of evidence-based programs and policies that are replicable, scalable, and sustainable.
6. Report biennially on progress throughout the decade from 2020 to 2030.
7. Stimulate research and innovation toward meeting *Healthy People 2030* goals and highlight critical research, data, and evaluation needs.
8. Facilitate development and availability of affordable means of health promotion, disease prevention, and treatment.